Parenting Power Struggle Handbook

Putting the pieces back together

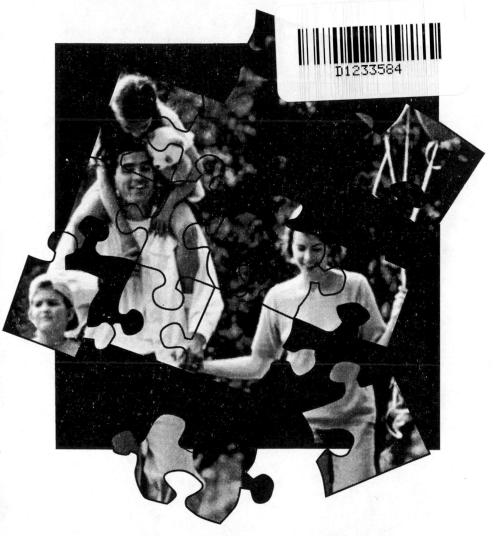

How to get out of power struggles NOW and avoid them in the future

by Timothy J. Hayes, Psy. D.

Printed in Victoria, Canada

National Library of Canada Cataloguing in Publication Data

A cataloguing record for this book that includes the U.S. Library of Congress Classification number, the Library of Congress Call number and the Dewey Decimal cataloguing code is available from the National Library of Canada. The complete cataloguing record can be obtained from the National Library's online database at: www.nlc-bnc.ca/amicus/index-e.html

ISBN: 1-4120-3624-0

TRAFFORD

This book was published *on-demand* in cooperation with Trafford Publishing. On-demand publishing is a unique process and service of making a book available for retail sale to the public taking advantage of on-demand manufacturing and Internet marketing. **On-demand publishing** includes promotions, retail sales, manufacturing, order fulfilment, accounting and collecting royalties on behalf of the author.

Suite 6E, 2333 Government St., Victoria, B.C. V8T 4P4, CANADA
Phone   250-383-6864   Toll-free   1-888-232-4444 (Canada & US)
Fax   250-383-6804   E-mail   sales@trafford.com
Web site   www.trafford.com
TRAFFORD PUBLISHING IS A DIVISION OF TRAFFORD HOLDINGS LTD.
Trafford Catalogue #04-1452   www.trafford.com/robots/04-1452.html

10   9   8   7   6   5

The Parenting Power Struggle Handbook

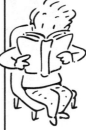

Table of Contents

**Table
of
Contents**

Design, layout and production by
Jill Sebenar Kaman, JSK Advertising Design
Spring Grove, IL • 815-675-2204

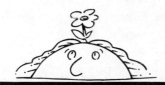

Chapter 1

The Parenting Power Struggle Handbook

Much of my work over the last twenty years has been with families where parents are asking me to help them gain control over their children. I tell them that I can't help them control their children. They are surprised to hear this but even more shocked when I tell them I don't think it is their job to control their children. I start with the observation, *I can't make anyone do anything they don't want to do.* I suggest that they have made the same observation and that is why they are coming to seek help.

You can't make anyone do anything they don't want to do.

Describing Your Job as a Parent.

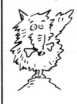

Often, when I then ask them to describe their job as a parent, they have trouble answering. So I suggest one way to look at the job of being a parent is to raise one's children to independence. This means that if the parents die, are disabled, or when the children reach adulthood, the children can care for and support themselves. Combine this with the observation, *you can't make anyone do anything they don't want to do,* and it may seem an impossible task. I suggest it is the parents' responsibility to **set rules, limits**, and **consequences** for their children and to provide them with the physical necessities of life. The parent's job is to watch children closely and to set and deliver consequences for their children's behavior. They provide positive consequences for behavior they feel will help their children learn to live independently and peacefully with others and negative consequences for behavior that they feel will hurt their children's chances for living independently and peace-fully. The parents are responsible for doing the *best job* they can *each day* to educate their children about what they think is going to help their children later in life. Parents do not receive credit for the successes of their children. The children work hard for their own achievements. The parents only get credit for their own behavior and the choices they make in how they raise their children. The children are then responsible for their behavior and their own successes and failures.

Discipline

In the past, parents often chose to spank or hit their children to let them know when they were behaving inappropriately. Currently, spanking and/or hitting is considered abusive punishment by many. It is important to have an effective substitute for spanking, hitting, swearing and/or screaming. The power struggle model and the systems of rules and consequences that parents develop for their children replace these forms of physical punishment for inappropriate behavior. Parents need to pay attention to their children's behavior and stay focused on the consequences that they, as parents, *can* control. This way they can choose to be as lenient or as strict as they want to be **without the use of physical punishment and without giving up their authority and letting their children run the household.**

What is a Power Struggle?

Most power struggles happen when: *we are trying to get someone to do something they don't want to do.*

When we have most of our energy focused on things we cannot control and very little energy focused on things we can control, **we leave ourselves open to a power struggle.**

We think we can control or have the right to control many things we actually cannot. We need to learn to separate those things we *can* control from those things we *cannot* control. This takes practice and it may require some outside advice.

We get angry at a traffic jam. We get furious when someone does not do something we tell them to do. We are upset when our car doesn't start or when it rains on a day we had planned to go to a baseball game.

Much of the time, all we really can control is our own behavior.

When dealing with our children, we have the luxury of controlling our own behavior and a variety of things related to the family household, clothing, recreational material, money, etc. When these things are correctly identified and used in a creative and structured way, they can be very useful in making our lives happier, safer and less stressful.

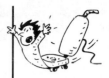

Power struggle and the car!

Many times parents come to me in a panic because their child will soon be old enough to have a driver's license. They are concerned because the teenager has not yet shown that he can be responsible for his behavior. I tell the parents to be glad that their child is approaching this milestone. The parents have control over whether or not the teenager gets a license and whether he or she keeps it. The parents own the car. The use of the car should be controlled by the owner. They now have control over something which may motivate their teenager to behave in a responsible manner. It is the parents' obligation to see that their children do not receive freedoms without first being able to live up to the responsibilities that come with those freedoms.

You are feeling out of control because you have focused most of your energy on something you cannot control.

How to Identify a Power Struggle.

Identifying a power struggle is not difficult. It is an **emotional response.** It is the feeling of frustration that leads to a sense of being out of control with a situation. The following steps will help you learn to identify a power struggle.

1. When you have a problem with someone, you put some energy into trying to solve it. When it doesn't get resolved, you feel **frustrated**. At this point, you **might** be in a power struggle.

2. When you try a second time to solve the problem by putting more energy into it and again you're not successful, you become **more frustrated**. At this point, you are **probably** in a power struggle.

3. When you try a third time, putting an even greater amount of energy into solving the problem and you

are still not successful, you begin to feel **out of control.** At this point, you are **DEFINITELY** in a power struggle. It is the feeling of being out of control that is the key to knowing when you are in a power struggle with someone else.

Begin by shifting the focus of your energy from those things you cannot control to those things you *can* control. Once you have correctly defined what you *can* control, you will immediately feel more *in* control! This will be true even if the problem isn't solved exactly the way you wanted.

You will be more relaxed because you are no longer feeling out of control. You will think more clearly and act more wisely.

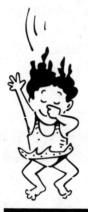

It is absolutely necessary to correctly identify and define the things around you that you *can* and *cannot* control. This takes practice!

We will all have times when we are under so much stress, or so tired, or so distracted that we fall back into old habits. At these times, we can only hope to catch ourselves when we begin to feel out of control. Then we can take a step back and shift the focus of our energy to things we *can* control and get back on track.

Take the Challenge!

First
Challenge yourself to recognize when you are feeling out of control.

Second
Challenge yourself to correctly identify what you can and cannot control.

Third
Challenge yourself to be creative in using the things you *do* have control over to make your life more safe, more sane, and more enjoyable.

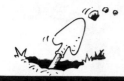

Chapter 2

How to Get Out of a Power Struggle and How to Avoid It.

Ask someone to do something once. Wait a reasonable period of time. If the other person has not followed your request, *begin to focus your attention and your energy on a list of what you will do if they do not comply*. No matter how simple this sounds, it contains real power. Using the following set of rules when making your list will magnify its power. All four rules must be used at the same time for it to work.

Rule One:
Make sure every item you put on your list is something you CAN do.

Rule Two:
Be sure that every item you put on your list is something you WILL do.

Rule Three:
Each of the things you put on your list must be something you can do WITHOUT STRONG EMOTION.

Rule Four:
Every item on your list must NOT be something that is designed to get the other person to do what YOU want. *It must be designed to make things better for YOU no matter what the other person does*.

It's important to note, in order for this to work...

Everyone must be treated with equal respect at all times.

If you follow these simple rules and do it with respect it can be used with anyone at anytime including your spouse, children, friends, boss, or employees. While this method will not magically succeed in getting you everything you want out of life, it will help you get more with less frustration.

Everyone should be treated with equal respect at all times.

The harder you work to match what you say with what you do, the more people will begin to believe you.

One of the most important tools a person has in his life is his credibility. By this I mean, *how easy it is for someone to believe that a person will do what they say.* There are two important things to do if you want to build your credibility. The first is to match what you say with what you do. The second is to be careful not to promise things you cannot or will not deliver.

If my child asks me if we can go to the pool tomorrow and I simply say, *Yes*, I am setting myself up for possible problems. What happens if it is raining the next day or my child doesn't behave and I say we aren't going to the pool? I will hear, "But dad, you promised.", or "But dad you said we could go. You lied!"

To avoid all of this, I need to be more specific with my answer. So when my child asks if we can go to the pool tomorrow, I can say, "We will be able to go if you are well behaved, the weather is good, and we have the time." This answer takes more thought but it pays many times over in the way it builds and protects my credibility.

In my experience, it has been my credibility that has been my greatest tool in dealing with people. No one is perfect and no one can always make good on everything they say but the more energy one puts into developing one's credibility the greater the pay off.

On those rare occasions when people come back and report that the power struggle model has not worked for them, we usually find that the people are lacking in consistency and/or credibility. They say things that they cannot or will not do, hurting their credibility.

Another problem I find is people expecting instantaneous results. When this doesn't happen, we almost always discover that these people have a history of telling people things that they either cannot or will not do. In these cases, all that is needed is time to prove their reliability and build their credibility. The longer you work at matching what you say with what you do, the more people begin to believe you. It takes time to correct a behavior pattern and to change people's perception of you. This will happen more quickly if you make the change promptly and consistently. It also helps to announce the change. You might start by saying, 'I know that I haven't in the past, but...'

Make a List, Follow These Simple Rules, Solve a Problem!

Rule One: Every item you put on your list must be something you CAN do.

This means you will not be prevented from doing each item on the list physically, legally, morally, financially, or in any other way. For example, don't tell your teenager that if she doesn't pick up her room you will pick her up with your little finger and throw her to Nebraska. If you know you can't physically do it, *don't say it.* Don't tell your teenager that if he doesn't pick up his room you will move to another house and he will have to live in the current house alone. Unless you have enough money to buy and maintain two households and legally the child is old enough to live alone, *don't say it.* This applies to any restrictions you may use. **If you can't do it, don't put it on your list.** Each time you put something on your list that you cannot do, you make it more difficult for the people around you to believe that you mean what you say.

Rule Two: Every item you put on your list must be something you WILL do.

This means you will actually do whatever you put on your list. Consistency is essential here. It is the only way to make yourself believable. For example, you shouldn't say to your teenager that if they don't pick up their room you will: 1. Pick up all the things on the floor and give them to the Salvation Army. 2. You will make their curfew one half hour earlier each night so that they

If you put it on your list and you don't do it, you damage your credibility.

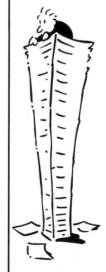

7

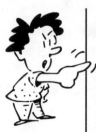

Strong emotion is the quickest way to mess up any plan to make things better.

have time to pick up their room so that it will never get dirty again. 3. You will run around the outside of their school three times, naked. Then, when they don't pick up their room, you take all their things to the Salvation Army and make their curfew a half an hour earlier each night. WAIT! If you didn't intend to run around the outside of their school three times, naked, you shouldn't have put it on your list. You say you intended to but your child begged you not to saying it would be too embarrassing. It doesn't matter how embarrassing it is. *If you put it on your list and you don't do it,* **you damage your credibility.**

Rule Three: Every item you put on your list must be something you can do WITHOUT STRONG EMOTION.

Strong emotion is the quickest way to mess up any logical system. Before you can get any productive work done, you need to manage strong emotions. This does not mean a parent should not get mad if the children play football in the living room and break an expensive piece of furniture that has been in the family for years. It only means that before the parent decides what the consequences are going to be for bad behavior, the parent needs some time to cool off and think clearly so that the consequences fit the crime and are not based on the anger of the moment. Overly harsh punishment leads to the parent feeling guilty later, and increases the chances that the consequence will not be enforced.

Another problem is, children enjoy pushing mom or dad's "hot buttons" regardless of the punishment. They will risk even greater punishment and loss of privileges for the payoff of witnessing an uncontrolled emotional response from their parents. No one knows exactly why, but everyone with children knows this happens.

Last but not least, if you use your emotions (and therefore your personality) to try to force people to do what you want, that part of your personality will not be available for developing and nurturing a relationship. If you use things you CAN control such as a consequence for undesirable behavior, then you are free to use your emotions and personality in a positive way to build a relationship with that person.

Rule Four: Every item you put on your list must NOT be something that is designed to get the other person to do what YOU want them to do. *It must be designed to make things better for YOU regardless of what the other person does.*

Most people have a hard time with this step. Remember that we began by observing that *you cannot make anyone do anything they don't want to do.* So if we get to Rule Four and say that we must cleverly design our lists to manipulate or force others to do what we want them to do, then we are being two faced.

All four rules must be used at the same time for it to work.

The first step toward success is to build your own credibility. Then people will have every reason to believe what you say.

Don't Forget:
You can't make anyone do anything they don't want to do. **You should think of this as a law, like the law of gravity. We can accept it and work with it or spend our lives fighting against it.**

You can't make a three-year-old stop crying. You can't make a teenager pick up his or her room. You can't make your spouse keep dirty clothes off the bedroom floor. In each case, they will stop either when they are ready or when they decide it is better to stop than to face the consequences. There are natural consequences and imposed consequences. A natural consequence is something that happens automatically. For instance if you go out in the rain without a raincoat or umbrella the natural consequence is that you will get wet. If you fall down and scrape your knee the natural consequence is that you feel pain.

The first step toward success is to build your own credibility.

9

An imposed consequence is something that another person controls. If your boss tells you to be at work at 8:00 am and you choose to arrive at 9:00 am, your boss could impose the penalty of suspending you for a day or putting a written notice in your file. If your child is supposed to come home right after school but decides to go to a friend's house instead, you could impose the consequence of no television for the rest of the evening. Of course this will only work if you are there to supervise and make sure that your child does not watch television that evening. Consequences only work when they are enforced. *A consequence that you don't follow through on hurts your credibility.*

Pick Up Those Blocks!

One night, about five years after I had started teaching my patients about power struggles, I stayed home with our two children while my wife went to work. They wanted to play with their blocks before bed. I told them no because they never wanted to pick up the blocks when they were finished playing with them. They promised to pick up the blocks and so I agreed to get them out. After about 45 minutes, it was time to pick up the blocks. I had two baskets of laundry to fold and I still had to get them a snack, brush their teeth and read them a story before bed. I told them to start picking up the blocks. They began to move as slow as molasses in winter. I raised my voice and they moved even slower. At this point, I was getting agitated. I felt I must win this battle. I needed to teach my children to do what they had promised, otherwise they would learn to be disrespectful of authority, flunk out of high school, and live on the streets as bums. All because they would not pick up their blocks when told. I became convinced that this was a battle I had to win if I were to be a good parent.

In short order, I was a raving, red faced maniac, screaming through tightly clenched teeth, "Pick up those blocks!" I picked up a block and slapped it into the hand of our three-year-old. I folded his little fingers around the block and put his hand over the block box. I then unfolded his fingers, letting the block drop into the box. Then I placed another block in his hand and yelled that he should, "Put that block into the box along with all the rest of them, NOW!" Our child was frozen with a mixture of surprise and confusion. After a moment or two, he looked directly at me and slowly rotated his hand with the block in it. When his hand was facing the ground, he slowly opened his hand and allowed the block to fall to the floor, nowhere near the block box.

In that instant, I wanted to do two things: give him a spanking he wouldn't forget and give him a hug and a kiss. I didn't do either. Instead, I sat back and took a deep breath and realized I was out of control. Our three year old had told me loud and clear that I was focusing all my energy on something I couldn't control. For that I wanted to give him a hug and a kiss.

I started to fold the laundry and began to think of what I would tell my patients to do in this situation. I would tell them to *take a time out* and make a list of *the things they can control* and *the things they cannot control.* Then I would tell them to focus their attention on the things they can control and to make a plan based on those things.

I took another piece of laundry out of the basket and thought about what I could control. I have control over bedtime, snacks, stories and music. As I calmly folded more laundry, I told our children that if they could get all the blocks picked up by the time I folded all the laundry in the two baskets, they could have their regular bedtime snack, story and music to listen to as they fell asleep. But if all of the blocks were not picked up by the time I was done, they would go right to bed with nothing. They immediately started jumping around talking about what snack, story and tape they wanted. They put an occasional block into the box but most of the blocks did not get picked up. I put them right to bed. They cried when they realized they wouldn't have their normal bedtime routine. They cried while their teeth were being brushed and then cried themselves to sleep.

You can't make anyone do anything they don't want to do.

I tucked them into bed with a hug and a kiss. I told them I loved them and that I was sorry they didn't get the blocks picked up because I liked reading to them and I was going to miss that tonight. I reminded them that there is always tomorrow and hopefully the next time they would do what they were told, so that they could have a snack, a story and bedtime music. It took me two or three minutes to pick up the blocks and put them away, noting to myself that I would not be getting them out again anytime soon.

Analysis

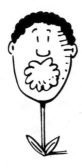

No matter how well practiced you are at avoiding power struggles, there might be times when you are tired or preoccupied and end up in the middle of an intense power struggle. Fortunately, once you recognize what has happened, it is possible to get out of it.

Our children and I took turns focusing our energy on things we had no control over. At first I had all my energy focused on making them pick up the blocks *(which they controlled)*. This left me feeling more and more frustrated. Next, our children focused all their energy on their snack and their story *(which I controlled)*, and not on picking up their blocks *(which they controlled)*. They could easily have picked up twice as many blocks in half the time it took me to fold the laundry. Instead, they spent all their energy talking about how they wanted their snack and story.

When I realized we were in a power struggle, I started following the four steps; I stopped feeling frustrated and angry. I was free to be a concerned parent and I could respond to their tears with empathy. I told them I knew they were unhappy. I was sad, too. I was sorry they didn't get the blocks picked up and I reminded them there would be another chance to do as they were told tomorrow.

I also listed only things I *could* and *would* do. I did not change the consequences for their behavior based on their level of tears. Once I had told them what I would do, *I followed through with every item on my list.*

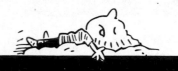

Battery-napppers Confronted!

When I was in graduate school, funds were very tight. I got tired of buying batteries for my pager so I bought a battery charger and kept it at home. It worked out beautifully until my wife and children discovered that toys and tape recorders would also work with rechargeable batteries. When I went to get a replacement battery for my pager, there were no batteries in the charger. I was angry. I told my wife I was angry. I told my children, (who were too young to be responsible for this kind of thing), I was angry. I went to the store and bought another package of batteries. I put one in the pager, hid the other one, and then *made a plan!* Once I cooled off, I talked to my wife. I told her everyone could use the battery charger as long as there was always a freshly charged battery left in it for my pager. If I went to the charger and there were no batteries when I needed them, I would use the extra battery I had hidden and then take the charger to work. Once there, it would be safe from prowling battery-nappers.

Analysis

In this example, I focused on the things I could control. My list included things I *could* and *would* do. I *could* take the battery charger to work because it had been purchased for that purpose, and I *would* take it to work if needed. I completed all four steps to avoid a power struggle. I had a conversation with my wife without getting upset (strong emotion). I talked to her without getting angry and yelling about her being irresponsible or not being concerned about my needs, etc. I was able to state firmly and calmly what I would do to make my life more sane and workable. I could relax because I did not have to monitor their behavior or constantly remind them to put batteries in the charger. I had established credibility with my family and they knew if I was without a fresh battery for my pager, I *would* take the charger to work.

The problem with doing something new is that it feels stiff and unnatural. To solve this problem, use this new plan consistently until it feels natural. When we all began to drive a car, there was so much to learn, it was difficult to keep everything straight. After years of practice, most of us are so comfortable with driving that we can be mentally distracted momentarily and still drive safely because the skills have become automatic.

The best time to learn to drive a car is when there is little or no traffic, in an open area and with no obstacles. The best time to decide what you might do in a power struggle is to think about it when you are calm and relaxed. Remember the last few power struggles you were involved in. Think about how you might have handled things differently to avoid one or end it more quickly. Eventually, when you find yourself in a similar situation, you can try out the things you have thought about. Gradually, you will build the habit of thinking in terms of *things you can control* and build the skill of making a plan based on that. There are three charts at the end of this booklet that may help you do this.

Think before you act.
When thinking about how to respond to a situation it is a good idea to take a deep breath and mentally rehearse what you want to say. Think of three people that you respect. Anytime you find yourself in an emotionally charged situation, stop and ask yourself, **"What would they do** in this situation? How is that different from what I might do?" Once you have those answers, ask yourself, "How might this effect the future? Is this likely to cause a positive change?"

Have you ever reacted like this?
Your sixteen-year-old asks for the car keys so that he can *hang out* with his friends. You look over at the kitchen sink, full of the dirty dishes he agreed to clean, and suddenly you see red! You can react immediately and start screaming things like, "I'm sick and tired of

giving and getting nothing back. Why can't you be more responsible about your chores? You are just a lazy, self-centered person and I'm never giving you the keys to the car again."

What just happened?

Try to think before you react. Tell your teenager you want to think about it. You can even go to another room if you are really angry. Then ask yourself these questions: **WWTD - What would they** (the three people I respect) **do?** What is the chance my child will do it right the *next time* because of what I say *this time*? Will I feel better for having said these things to my child after I've had a chance to calm down and think about it?

You may be surprised at the answers. One thing I can almost guarantee, you will do it differently if you give yourself the chance to think about what you are going to say.

The most important message a parent can give a child is that: **You have two parents that love you very much.** *This must be done with both words and actions.*

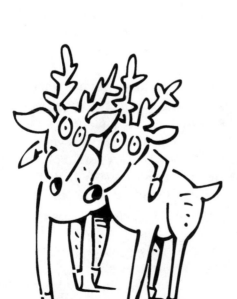

Chapter 3

Put the Power Struggle Model to Work for You!

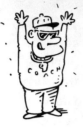

The power struggle model is just one part of a larger system that works to establish appropriate rules, limits, and consequences in your home, personal or professional life. Any plan established with the hope of success must follow certain guidelines. The following are some suggestions:

If whatever you are doing is not working, try something else.

How do you decide if something is working? You must continually reevaluate whether it is useful when it comes to discipline. An important guideline is how often you have to use a consequence. If you have to use it less often, it is having the desired effect. If you have to use it consistently or more and more often, it is not working; try something else.

Remember: discipline should immediately be followed by a hug and a parent telling the child, "I love you, even if I don't like what you did."

Repeatedly and consistently evaluate whether your efforts are succeeding based on things you can measure.

For example: if you tell your child that for every class where she shows improvement you will give her some money, this is too loose to be useful. You would need to be clear and tell her that for every D she improves to a C, you will give her $5, or for every test score above an 80% she can rent a video game over the weekend.

Never set a rule or consequence you cannot enforce.

If you won't be around to enforce the rule or consequence, don't set it. Suppose the children in the family are not doing well in school. The parents tell them they are not allowed to watch television until all of their homework is done each night. The children get home at least two hours before the parents, so they are able to watch television without the parents' knowledge. This rule is unenforceable. They should try something else.

You can't make anyone do anything they don't want to do.

Whenever possible, make consequences follow immediately after the undesired behavior.
The closer to the undesired behavior the greater the chance the consequence will be effective. If the child is too young or too much time has passed since the behavior occurred, it is best not to give a consequence. When this happens, tell the child what the consequence will be if it happens again. For example: if you move a dresser and find that someone has written on the wall, you have no way of knowing when it happened or who did it. Show the damage to the child or children and explain what will happen if this occurs again.

Try to *make the punishment fit the crime.*
A common way parents break this rule is to tell their children that if they don't eat their dinner they will not be able to go out to play, watch television, or pursue another type of recreation. The problem is that eating is not related to play. A better consequence for a child who chooses not to eat would be no dessert or snacks until the next scheduled meal. Another example of making the punishment fit the crime follows: one of my co-workers came home from work one day to find the house covered with graffiti. The following weekend, the culprit (her 14-year old son) was not allowed to do any-thing until he repainted the entire outside of the house. The chances are good that he won't repeat that behavior.

Try to set up a system that is more focused on positive reinforcement and positive consequences.
Think about what will motivate a child, adolescent, or adult. Be willing to accept the fact that different people will be motivated by different things. A work sheet at the end of this booklet will help you think about how to motivate positive behavior.

Look at the effectiveness of the system often.
The usefulness of consequences and rewards can, and does change frequently in life from one situation to the next. Be creative and think of each individual and

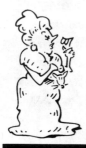

situation as a new place to practice your limit setting and evaluate the effectiveness of your choices.

Remember: Always, but especially if there has been a divorce or separation, one of the most important messages a parent can give a child is: *You have two parents that love you very much.* This must be done with both words and actions.

Building House Rules and Family Structure.

Discipline should be immediately followed by a hug and a parent telling the child that I love you even if I don't like what you did.

The basis of any household is structure. It may be informal and loose or formal and highly detailed. The way you set up your household is your choice. Establishing rules and their consequences makes it possible to create the kind of atmosphere you want. This always works best when the parents are communicating well and negotiate different points where they disagree.

There needs to be a set of rules for discipline in the house that BOTH parents agree upon and which are not argued about in front of the children.

Parents will have different opinions about how certain situations should be handled and this is normal. Some of these can be negotiated to find a solution both parents support. Others will never be agreed upon. In these instances, the children will learn that when mom is with them, things work one way and when dad is with them, things work another way. Where a disagreement remains, the parent who starts working with the children should be the one to follow through and finish making the decision regarding reward or punishment.

Rules are needed to specify what action one parent should take if they don't like what their partner is doing with regards to disciplining the children. Some questions requiring discussion are:

1. How are the rules decided and when are they discussed?

2. What incidents are serious enough to make one break these rules?

If one parent is at home with the children and the other parent comes home, that parent needs to check things out with the parent who has been there, before making any decisions. If two parents are home and an incident occurs that needs attention, the first parent to act gets to work the problem through without interference from the other parent. The second parent may have comments to make but should wait until the parents can talk privately. The only reason to break the rules, would be *agreed upon exceptions* between the parents, such as immoral, illegal, or harmful behavior. It is usually helpful to have a code word or phrase that the parents agree upon ahead of time which they use to tell each other that the parents need a time-out to discuss the problem before it goes any further.

I frequently tell people to stop and consider whether it is worth the energy to fight with your partner about the way he or she handled something with the children. I warn them to choose their battles carefully because it takes a lot of energy and can put a lot of stress on the relationship. Think about the fact that if your partner were raising the children all by his or herself, the children would probably grow up to be a lot like them. This can't be all bad, after all, you chose this person to share your life.

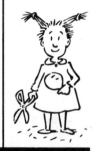

Who's in Charge?

When both parents are home and some form of limit setting or discipline is needed, who should do it? The answer depends on many things such as:

1. Who is the closest to the incident or actually involved in the incident?

2. Who has the time to deal with the incident?

3. Who is calm enough to deal with the incident without letting their emotions take control?

4. Who has a history of dealing with the children about this issue?

5. Who is most irritated or worried about the behavior in question?

When there is a step parent in the home, who should do the limit setting or discipline?

Usually, this list is exactly like the previous list. If there have been problems between the step parent and the children, the family needs to develop a policy about which parent will handle what discipline issues. This usually takes a great deal of effort. Many families have found that it is best for the biological parent to be responsible for their own child's discipline. This approach carries with it several complications and often it leaves a step parent feeling as though they have lost the adult authority in their own home. Using the power struggle model can help the step parent maintain their adult authority and still build a relationship with their step children.

Special notice to families who have been through a divorce or separation... One of the most important messages a parent can give a child is that **you have two parents who love you very much.** This must be shown with both words and actions. Any message other than this will put your child in the position of having to choose between two parents. This is a horrible thing to ask a child to do. It doesn't matter that your partner or ex-partner may say bad things about you; that's not something you can control. What you can control is whether or not you choose to put your children in the middle, pressuring them, either directly or indirectly, to choose between their parents. The most healthy thing you can do for your children is to give them the message that no matter how both parents may disagree about how to raise their children and whether or not the parents can learn to live peacefully together, *they still love their children in their own way, the best way they know how.*

Blended Families/Step Parents

One of the biggest problems with blended families, or families with step parents, is that the step parent tries to discipline a step child before there is a solid relationship established between the step parent and the step child. When this happens, the next most common mistake is for the step parent to try and force or manipulate the step child to do what he or she wants them to do. This cuts off any chance for the step parent to build a relationship with the child.

This is often complicated by the step parent's own emotional needs to feel accepted or important in the new family structure. I have run across this problem with biological parents as well. When the parent becomes too focused on feeling liked or loved by the child, they are focused on something they have no control over, namely the child's emotions and reactions.

You can't make anyone do anything they don't want to do.

Once this happens the parent or step parent begins to get frustrated and often gets overly emotional. This of course simply disrupts the logic of any discipline they are trying to apply and makes it harder for them to build a relationship with the child. I used to tell people that if my children did not tell me "I hate you", or "I don't like you" at least twice a week, then I am probably not doing my job as a parent. The preferred way to respond to this kind of statement is for me to say either, "I know you're feeling that way at this moment, but it won't last", or, "Well I'm sorry you feel that way, because I love you.". The reality is that if you do your job well as a parent, your children will either choose to love you or not. There is nothing you can do about this. The good part about this is that human beings have an incredibly strong tendency to love their parents no matter how many things their parents do that the child doesn't like.

But I Want My Child to Love Me!

I strongly believe that it is not my job to make my children love me, but to do the best I can at loving them and sending them clear messages when I feel they are doing things that I feel will help them later on in life

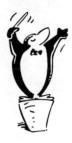

(encouragement and rewards), and clear messages when I feel they are doing things that will hurt them later in life (discipline and consequences). If I am able to keep my focus on these things, and the love I have for them, our nature as human beings will take care of the rest. Children will naturally love their parents and want their parents to love them, even though they get angry at their parents. If you, as a parent, are worried that your children won't love you, you may need help with your own insecurity.

A well-designed family structure can help a family resolve many difficulties and avoid others completely. A book on parenting skills or a therapist may be needed to gain the objective distance and experience to find a solution to the problem. I believe that one of the hardest things anyone can do is join two families under one roof. All families have problems making decisions about discipline. If you are having problems in this area, do some research, look for a support group, or get professional help. Whether you are using professional or nonprofessional help, please make sure that:

1. The person or group you are using knows what they are doing.
2. You, or you and your spouse, are comfortable with the person or group.

If you don't feel that either of these are true, the therapy or treatment will not be helpful. I have listened to many stories over the years in which the parents went to fully licensed and credentialed professionals and received advice that the parents were not comfortable using. Don't be afraid to seek a second or third opinion and above all else, trust your *gut feeling* about the person and the advice you are receiving.

Guilt

Parents who start to work on problem patterns with their children sometimes feel guilty about the *harm* they may have done to their children. I tell them that they can either focus on the past, which they cannot control, or focus on their actions today, which they can control. If they choose the second option, I tell them to rejoice in the fact that if they make the appropriate changes they will be giving their children one of the most important gifts their children will ever receive. *The gift of showing your children that it is never too late to learn and change and grow into the kind of person that you want to be.* Guilt is often a very strong emotion; so strong that it is necessary to have it under control before deciding how to respond to your children. Otherwise you will ruin any good, logical plan you hope to have in place to build strong relationships with your children. Guilt is only useful if it motivates people to change undesired behavior. If guilt is not motivating a person to change a harmful or unproductive behavior then it usually keeps them locked in an unproductive pattern of self criticism.

Trust is a gift that people give to others!

Forgiveness and Trust

Often my work with families brings up the issue of forgiveness and trust. What do we do when someone has lied to us or treated us badly and we no longer trust them? I was originally taught that people had to earn someone's forgiveness and trust. I even worked for years helping families draw up contracts that detailed what an adolescent or a spouse would have to do in order to *earn* someone's forgiveness and trust.

The problem with this was that sometimes it worked but many times it did not. Many times the person would perform all the tasks asked of them in the contract, only to learn that the other person still did not forgive them or trust them. Often the whole idea of the contract was used to suggest that the person who had *lost* the trust, was only doing what the contract said in order to *earn back* the trust and that they really did not *mean it*. This meant that they would probably break that contract as soon as the other person forgave them and trusted them again.

My observation is that forgiveness and trust are gifts that people give others when they want to give them. It has nothing to do with whether people have earned it.

I have watched people trust complete strangers. On the other hand I have watched people get tricked, fooled and lied to numerous times by someone they know and then continue to trust them.

I encourage people to be more responsible with their own trust and forgiveness since these are gifts they can give or withhold as they choose.

In my opinion, it does not make sense to forgive or trust someone for doing something seriously wrong unless they have done the following four things:

1. admitted that what was done was wrong,
2. made a genuine apology,
3. made amends for any harm caused in any way,
4. taken concrete steps to change things in an effort to ensure that they won't repeat the mistake.

I tell people that they should develop their own standards of who to trust and when. I remind them that they can choose to forgive someone and still decide not to trust them because they haven't demonstrated that they are trustworthy. I suggest that people should apply these standards with less regard for their emotions, and more regard for the results. For instance, if the standard is set so that a person gets three chances, *three strikes and you're out,* then it doesn't matter if the person who strikes out is my friend or my son or my partner. I still don't trust them because they have proven that they are not trustworthy. When I choose to give my trust to someone who has proven, by their actions, that they are not trustworthy, then I am to blame for any harm or problem that results when they don't live up to that trust. I should have known better because they have already demonstrated that they are not trustworthy.

On the other hand, I can still refuse to trust someone who has betrayed my trust several times even though they have worked hard to prove themselves trustworthy. This, however, would be my loss because I am keeping the relationship from growing because I am not willing to risk being disappointed again.

It is a choice people make when they decide to forgive and to trust. Forgiveness and trust are not things to be earned, but gifts each of us decide to give or withhold.

As parents we need to decide if we want our children to learn that people will trust them no matter what they do. If this is the case, we should trust our children no matter how they perform. If we want our children to learn that most people will only trust them if they have shown they can act in a trustworthy manner, then we should withhold our trust until our children have demonstrated that they are trustworthy.

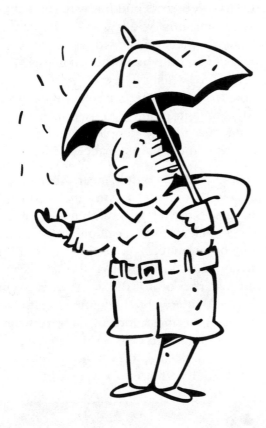

Chapter 4

Boundaries

Personal bound- aries are messages you give that tell people how you feel about things you think are not accept- able.

One of the most useful concepts I have encountered is that of personal and family boundaries. In general this means that anything you say or do lets other people know what you think is acceptable and not acceptable. This includes the way you express yourself when you are angry; whether you get angry when it is appropriate; whether you are comfortable expressing positive emotions such as love or joy; whether you confront people who are, in your opinion, wrong and whether you do this respectfully; the way you dress and the way you talk; whether you swear and how you react when others swear around you; whether you use words like please and thank you and what you do when others don't use those words; whether you are willing to leave a situation when it is unacceptable to you or whether you will passively accept things that, in your opinion, are wrong. These are the types of things that tell the people around you what you feel is acceptable and what is unacceptable.

Creating boundaries within a family means that anything that is said and done communicates to other people that members of this group are a family. Within a family, this may include things such as whether phone calls are taken during meal time or after a certain hour at night. It may also include the hours of the day that visitors are welcome in the home and whether or not the family engages in activities as a group that are clearly defined as family activities. Examples of this might include going to religious or spiritual services on certain days, or designating a weeknight or weekend day as a time when the family works or plays together with few, if any, exceptions.

Generational Boundaries

An extremely important concept in the family structure is the idea of a *Generational Boundary.* This can be defined as those things that are said and done that clearly communicate that the parents are on one level and the children are on a completely different level within the family structure. This is important for a variety of reasons. It allows for a clear definition of authority which is important for a family structure to operate effectively. The Generational Boundary is often defined by the fact that certain topics are for discussion by adults only; certain topics are for discussion by adults and proclamation to children; certain topics are fair game for children and adults alike; and certain topics are for parents and children to discuss only in relation to how they relate to the children's life. For example, in most families it is not viewed as appropriate for the parents to talk to the children about the parents' sex-lives, but it is important for the parents to educate their children about sex and how they integrate that part of their lives into healthy relationships. Each family needs to decide what these rules will be. There can be a great deal of variation from one family to another. As long as the rules are part of a well thought out and consistently applied family structure, they have a good chance of working out well for that family.

Bound-aries are a useful way to let others know what you think is accept-able and not accept-able.

Personal Boundaries

Personal boundaries are likewise established by an individual with everything he or she says and does that helps other people know what that person feels is appropriate and inappropriate. This can be something as subtle as a facial expression when someone tells a joke that you feel is in bad taste. It could also be as dramatic as abruptly leaving a room, or taking physical action to defend yourself or your property. Personal boundaries are established by things as simple as the way you dress, or your tone of voice as you respond to someone saying or doing something that you find unacceptable. The more you pay attention to what you are doing and the messages it gives, the easier it will be to set the limits or boundaries you want to set.

27

Chapter 5

Bottom Line Rules

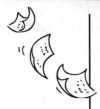

There are seven *bottom line rules or observations* I use when doing therapy with people.

1. If whatever I am doing is not working, I need to try something else.

2. Blame is a luxury item; it will never lead to a productive or constructive resolution of a problem.

3. I can't make *anyone* do *anything* they don't want to do.

4. I can only be *responsible for* and *control* my own emotions and reactions. I cannot control or be responsible for the emotions and reactions of anyone else.

5. My greatest strengths and assets will also, at times, be my greatest weaknesses and liabilities.

6. When I ignore or deny the negative emotions and experiences in life, I cut off an equal amount of positive emotions and experiences.

   The best way to smother the intimacy in a relationship is to avoid conflict and confrontation. If you don't know how to turn confrontation in to resolution, LEARN!

7. Each day I am alive I become more and more like my parents.

   Your children will grow up to be more like you than anything you will ever tell them you want them to be.

The good news is, you get both good and bad traits from your parents and if this is recognized you can choose to play up the good and minimize the not so good parts of who your parents were. So if you don't like what you see coming out of your children, *focus more energy on try-ing to become the kind of person you want <u>them</u> to be.*

We don't like to think about how we are becoming more and more like our parents as we get older, but if we accept this fact then we can start to change the inappropriate behavior that is affecting our children.

If we as parents can accept that we will be more like our parents every day and that our children will be more like us every day, then we will be able to concentrate on what we are doing, as it happens, and choose those actions that will help us be the kind of person we want to be.

One of the most important things to remember as a parent is that your children will grow up to be like you no matter what you do. The next thing to remember is that your *actions* will be screaming at your children so loudly that they will not be able to hear your words. This is another way of saying that no matter what you tell your children to do *they will do what you do, rather than what you say.*

No matter what you tell your children you want them to be, they will grow up to be more like you than anything else.

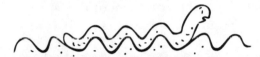

Some Common Problems When Using This Model

- Breaking one or more of the four *Power Struggle Rules*.

- Giving punishments that are too harsh, making it hard to follow through on them.

- Forgetting to tell someone that you respect them as a person and/or love them, despite their inappropriate behavior.

- Not choosing your battles carefully. Is this problem worth *fighting over?* Remember your priorities!

- Thinking that you can or should control things that you cannot.

- Setting rules you cannot or will not be around to enforce.

- Trying to take responsibility for another person's emotions or reactions.

- Focusing more on the negative and not enough on the positive aspects of a person and their behavior.

Chapter 6

Behavior Monitoring and Limit Setting

Time Out

Too many people do not understand the idea of a time-out. They either use it as a punishment, or use it as a way to avoid dealing with an unpleasant situation with their child. A time-out is not meant as a punishment but as a time for the child to decide how to act. It should come after the child has been told that their actions will lead to a punishment or consequence if they don't change their behavior. This is a time for the child and/or the adult to defuse their intense emotions. It is a cooling off period and should be used when it is likely to lead to a more calm discussion of the problem or the consequences that need to be given for a problem behavior. There are times when a 'time-out' is not appropriate because it simply is not a strong enough message about how the parent feels about the child's behavior. There are many times when it is more appropriate to give a consequence such as an earlier bedtime, or the loss of part of an allowance, or the loss of the use of a toy for a specific time. This will depend on how strong a message the parent wishes to send. There are times when a time-out is appropriate and may be all that is needed for the child to calm down and avoid further consequences. However if the child refuses to calm down and take a time-out, then it is appropriate for the parent to impose a further consequence.

Pestering and Badgering

It is common for parents to return after trying to set some limits and state that they did not give in to their child, but that the child made them miserable with pestering and badgering for hours. It is important to remember that anything your child says or does is a behavior that can be labeled as acceptable or unacceptable. It is the parents' responsibility to give consequences for those behaviors. Since many of the rules and limits that parents set are not going to be popular with their children, parents should expect that there will be questions, complaining, whining or maybe even tantrums. The parents should be prepared with consequences for these behaviors as well.

Sometimes parents say they don't want to punish their child for simply asking questions. I ask them to think about what would happen if they were at work and asked for a day off and their boss told them 'no'. Then over the next several hours they asked their boss repeatedly to defend her decision and explain why they could not have the day off. Then after hours of constant questioning while neither they nor their boss were able to be very productive, they began to get angry with their boss for not giving them the answer they wanted. If this is not a behavior that will benefit your child as an adult, you should be giving consequences for it when they are children.

Often the most useful consequence is an exaggeration of the very thing the child is complaining about. For example:

Child: "Mom can we rent a video game today?"

Parent: "No dear. Not today."

Child: "Oh please, Mom. Please. Pretty please with sugar on top."

Parent: "No dear! Not today!"

Child: "Oh Mom, why not? You let Larry rent a video game when he wants to. Come on, Mom! Please! I promise I won't bother you all day if you just let me rent one game."

At this point something should be done by the parent to set a limit. But often the parent repeats the same thing they have already said and gets the same result.

Parent: "No! You can't rent a video game!"

Child: "Oh come on, Mom, there's nothing else to do. Please! What about how you said last week that this weekend we would do something fun? Come on, you promised!"

If whatever you are doing is not working, try something else.

31

Parent: "I said no and I mean NO!"

Child: "This isn't fair! You promised! What if I paid for it with my own money? Then would it be all right?"

Parent: "No. I am not going to drop everything and drive you to the video store. I have work to do."

Child: "Oh come on, it won't take long. Please! I'll be good, I promise I won't ask you for anything else all day."

*If this sounds familiar, please reread it and notice how many times the parent in this example is saying the same thing and getting the same results. When using **the power struggle model,** a person only says something a certain way once, then the next time something needs to be said, it should be changed to focus on what the person will do if others don't do as they are asked.*

Try this:

Child: "Mom, can we rent a video game today?"

Parent: "No dear. Not today."

Child: "Oh, please Mom. Please. Pretty please with sugar on top."

Parent: "No dear! Not today! And if you ask me again, you won't get a video game tomorrow or the next day either. Now go play a game or read a book and don't ask me again unless you want to lose something else."

This example is much shorter. Therefore, it is much less frustrating for the parent and the child. The child can choose to keep asking, pestering or badgering, but there will be consequences of increasing severity as it continues. That would be the child's choice.

Another example:

Child: "Dad, I know you said I had to be home by ten but the guys are going out after the game and asked me to go. Can I be home by eleven instead?"

Dad: "No son. It is a school night and your curfew is ten o'clock."

Child: "Aw, but Dad, you always make me come home earlier than all my friends and it isn't fair. How about if I promise to be home by ten forty-five?"

Dad: "Nine-thirty!"

Child: "But my curfew is ten. You just said. How about ten-thirty?"

Dad: "Now it's nine! Care to try for eight-thirty?"

I don't mean to say by this example that parents should never negotiate with their children and never explain things to their children. There is a time and a place for everything. I don't believe it is ever a good thing to negotiate in the middle of a discussion for which there is already a rule and a decision has been made by the parent. When negotiation happens at times like this, it means the parent is most likely letting themselves be manipulated by the child.

The power struggle model makes things better for you regardless of what other people choose to do.

Counting

Many people have used the idea of counting to two or three or five to let the child know that they are close to getting a time-out or a consequence. Anyone who has worked with this idea knows that if you count to ten before giving a consequence or a time-out, your children will learn not to respond until you get to nine. If you count to three, your children will learn not to respond until two and a half. It is not unusual for two people who say they will count to three to get two very different responses from their children. The one parent may complain that the children always wait until after they have counted to three before doing anything. While the other person in the house rarely has to get to two before the children respond. It takes a little questioning to discover that the person who does not get a response until after they have counted to three has a habit of getting to three and then warning the child that they will lose a privilege or get a consequence. On the other hand, the person who gets a response on or before counting to two, usually gives a consequence immediately upon reaching a count of three. Often this person will say, "That's one...That's two... Now you have lost a privilege." Quickly the child learns that if they wait until the parent has said the word *three*, it is already too late.

Behavior Modification is Different From the Power Struggle Model

Behavior modification provides rewards after desired behavior and punishment after undesired behavior.

The following is a brief description of behavior modification to clarify how it is different from the power struggle model. For more details on how to set up a behavior modification plan, one should consult with a therapist, or get a book on behavior modification programs from the library.

Behavior modification is the planned arrangement of rewards and consequences in an effort to motivate someone to change their behavior. This is done by using a reward immediately after a desired behavior, and a negative consequence, or punishment immediately after an undesired behavior. In this system things are only called rewards if they increase the behavior that they follow, and things are only called punishments or negative consequences if they decrease the behavior that they follow.

Some Parents want to give consequences but can't think of any or can't afford to give the child a dollar each time they act appropriately, etc. One good way around this is to use a graph, chart or a token system that will let the parent and the child mark progress toward a goal.

Let's say that the child has been having trouble with a certain behavior such as picking on a sibling. This child would like to attend a party at school in three weeks. The parent can have the child make a chart that will be used to show days of acceptable behavior and days of unacceptable behavior. Then the parent can decide how many days of good behavior are going to be needed for the child to be able to attend the party at school. The progress can be marked daily or throughout the day, depending upon how detailed you make the chart.

Some families use the idea of a thermometer and give the child a strip of red for each good day or half-day of acceptable behavior. Then the child can watch the red line rise to the point where she has earned the privilege of going to the party.

In this situation the parent needs to be certain that they are the only ones that mark the chart and they may need to make sure that they use a special marker that only they possess. Or they may use their own signature or initials which can't be copied by a child who is overly anxious to see positive progress on the chart.

The options for the younger children include more immediate rewards like snacks and treats. For those that need more frequent reinforcement you can have them earn points which they trade in for snacks or treats. This can be tracked with slips of paper or pieces of a building toy like Legos. Each time the child earns another point for good behavior they are given another little Lego piece. Then at regular intervals they can trade their Legos in for a snack, or save them for a larger reward later in the day. Any system like this needs to be more focused on the positives than the negatives, however the child could also lose some Lego pieces for inappropriate behavior.

It should be noted that with any system like this, the *rewards* have to be evaluated frequently to make sure that they are valuable to the person gaining them. The *system* also needs to be evaluated frequently to make sure it's working – the undesired behaviors are happening *less* frequently and the desired behaviors are happening *more* frequently. There needs to be a feeling on the part of the parent that the effort it takes to set rules and give consequences and rewards is worth the result they are seeing in the child's behavior. The child should be sharing increasing responsibility for their behavior and its consequences as the child gets older. This will build a sense of competence in the child and ensure that they are better prepared to function in the world as they enter adulthood.

Rewards should be valued by the person getting them, to motivate them to change undesired behavior.

*Parents
need to
do things
that
aren't
always
easy
to send
a clear
message
to their
children
of what
is the
right
thing
to do.*

To illustrate an example of the difference between behavior modification and *the power struggle model* consider the following: if you ask your child to pick up their room and they don't do it, you may employ a behavior modification technique by saying that if the child picks up their room they can earn extra allowance or a video game, or they may refuse and lose an item or treat that they would normally get. *The power struggle model* suggests that if you tell your children to pick up their room by a certain time (because it's so messy *you* can't stand it), you will go into their room with a large garbage bag and pick up everything that is not where it belongs. The room will be clean and you will feel better. Then you can decide whether to donate those items to charity or hold them for a week, giving your child a chance to earn them back, or just throw it all away to teach your children that if they cannot take care of their belongings they will lose them.

Swearing

Some families find that they have a problem with inappropriate language or swearing in the house after the children reach a certain age and perhaps are exposed to it at school. One of the ways some families deal with this is to have a jar in the kitchen where *all* family members have to put a dime or quarter in the jar every time they swear or say words that are unacceptable, as defined by the parents. In most cases the parents find that they are also putting dimes or quarters in the jar for saying things that are not acceptable. Then at regular intervals the family can take the money in the jar and either donate it to a charity or use it for a family outing to promote better communication among the family. This could be a dinner at a restaurant, a trip to the zoo, a round of miniature golf, renting a video or ordering pizza so they can stay home together and play games one evening. In short, it should be any activity in which the family will interact with each other. This is a way of rewarding the family as a group for working to stop swearing.

Families today often find that with their hectic schedules they have difficulty getting the children to bed at the same time every day. They have difficulty having meals at a regular time or getting up at the same time in the morning. This is especially difficult on younger children. Many families notice marked improvement in their children's disposition when they start scheduling a standard, and usually earlier, bedtime as well as a morning rise time for their children *and stick to it.* Once this is done, the parents have created yet another set of consequences they can use to show their children how strongly the parents disapprove or approve of certain behaviors. Children can earn later bedtime or earlier bedtime, etc.

If the children have an established bedtime of 8:00 p. m. on weekdays and 9:00 on Friday and Saturday nights, then the parents can use an earlier bedtime as a consequence for inappropriate behavior during the day but especially during the evening hours. It is usually good to start with fifteen minute or half hour increments. A parent may tell a child that if they don't stop arguing they will go to bed 15 or 30 minutes early. This is usually looked at by the child as a form of torture. In reality, if the child is irritable and unable to behave properly, it may well be that he or she is tired and so the consequence is not only a punishment but also a solution to the child's fatigue.

There have been times when the parents I have worked with have sent their children to bed more than an hour early when they first try to use *the power struggle model,* and this type of consequence. It is because the children don't believe the parents will enforce the consequence and so they keep acting up until they have earned an earlier and earlier bedtime. When this happens, it is suggested that the child be supervised from outside the room so that the parent is sure the child is not doing anything other than lying quietly in bed or perhaps reading quietly.

Sticking to a schedule helps improve a child's disposition.

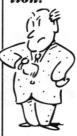

Trust your gut feeling about what is safe and how to act to protect you and your children.

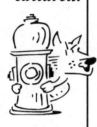

Again, when tantrums and crying and other forms of acting out occur, these need to be seen as separate behaviors that may require additional consequences. If the child is acting out in a way that might be harmful to himself or others or damaging property, I suggest that the parents seek professional advice on how to handle the situation in a way that will keep everyone safe and sane.

Over the years I have worked with many parents who have reached the point where they felt like they were prisoners in their own home. In one way or another they did not feel safe or they did not feel that their children were safe because of some pattern of behavior by one or more of the children or parents in the house. In these cases I always caution that people should consider safety first. People need to learn to trust their own *gut* feelings about what is safe and how to act in a way that will protect them and their children. If anything they do or any advice they receive results in things getting worse or more violent or in any way more scary or harmful, they should follow their own instincts to keep people safe and get additional outside help as soon as possible. Behavior can always be worked on at a later date as long as everyone is healthy and safe.

More Serious Offenses

Since my work as a probation officer from 1974-1976, I have been dealing with families who are experiencing problems with the law. I am often asked by parents how to deal with a child or teenager doing something illegal. There have been many times over the years when parents have found stolen goods in their house, or received information from someone that their child was involved in illegal activity. This often leads to a call to the psychologist. In these cases I ask the parents what message they want to send to their child.

I tell them that if they want their child to know that the child can break the law and their parents will lie for them and protect them from the consequences, then they should not report the offense. On the other hand, if they want their child to understand that there are consequences for our actions, they need to do something.

The parents may not always agree with the laws but they are subject to obey them or pay the consequences just like everyone else. The parents need to *do* things to get this message across to their child. This may mean turning in their own child to the police. It may mean offering the child the chance to change their behavior dramatically and make amends for any damage they have done. If the child does not choose to follow the rules and guidelines for making amends that the parents suggest, then the parents have no option but to turn the child over to the authorities and let their child deal with the consequences of their actions.

I often hear complaints from the parents that this will mean a great hardship for the family because of trips to court and the probation officer and the fact that the child might have to pay a fine or must pay restitution ordered by the court. My only response is that if the parent knows it is the right thing to do there is simply no excuse for not doing it. No matter how difficult it is, if you know it is the right thing to do for your child and for the situation, you either do it or face the consequences. One immediate consequence will be that the parent will teach the child by example, that they only do the right thing when it is convenient, or when it doesn't cost much.

Another consequence might be that the child gets caught by someone at a later date and then tells people that her parents knew about this activity for some time. This may result in a charge being brought against the parent for neglect or abuse or for encouraging an illegal activity by their child. I have had the unpleasant experience of watching loving parents who thought they were protecting their children, brought up on charges for contributing to the delinquency of a minor because they did nothing when they had evidence that their child was breaking the law.

I frequently have to ask parents whether they would rather have their child face charges as a juvenile for a first offense, or face charges as an adult for multiple

Parents who rescue their children as teenagers lose that ability once they become adults.

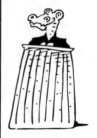

When someone has broken a rule, it is very impor- tant that they know what will happen if they do it again.

offenses. The reason I ask this is because I have watched many young people over the years *get rescued* by mom and/or dad with the result that they learn to expect to be rescued again and again. The problem is that while some people have the time, money and inclination to *rescue* their children while they are young, they lose this ability once the person is being prosecuted as an adult. This comes as a rude awakening to both the *child* and *the parent* but only when it is too late to change.

On many occasions the parents I have worked with have used the fact that they have evidence that their child has broken a law to motivate their child to begin to follow the rules of the house and the city and state. The way to do this is to formulate some new rules and consequences which they enforce and the child agrees to abide by. The only option for the child accepting the rules and consequences is that the parents *will* report what they know about their child's illegal activities to the police. I always caution parents to consult a lawyer or a law officer to learn about their rights and their responsibilities and liabilities before offering to with- hold information about a crime. Depending on the situation it may not be possible for the parents to withhold information about the incident without leaving themselves open to charges of neglect or contributing to the delinquency of a minor, or even obstruction of justice, or harboring a fugitive. I always suggest that parents arm themselves with as much solid information as they can before they decide what to tell their children. This will help the parents avoid telling their children something that the parents cannot or will not be able to do.

After a Violation

Be Specific about Future Consequences
The most important thing to do once someone has broken a rule is to be specific about what will happen if they do it again. A very well dressed professional gentleman with his 17 year old daughter came to my office. Despite being a straight A student who had never given her parents much trouble, there were beer bottles left in the family car after she used it one evening. Both

parents were horrified and did not know what to do, so they ended up in the psychologist's office.

I asked repeatedly what would happen the next time this occurred. The man and his daughter just kept saying, "It won't happen again." As I continued to push the question, the daughter kept saying, "It won't happen again because he would kill me." I tried to get them to understand that I did not think for a minute that this father would harm his daughter. They admitted they did not believe that either. As a result, the *consequence* she feared was not real. I tried to get them to understand the importance of making the consequence more specific and concrete.

I suggested that this intelligent, young woman may act differently if she knew that the next time her parents suspected her of letting someone drink in the car, they would do the following:
1. revoke her license.
2. deny her the privilege of driving a family car permanently.

This would mean she would have to be old enough to buy her own car and responsible enough to earn money for a car and insurance before she drove legally again.

This would give new meaning to the decision she would be faced with the next time one of her friends begged her to give them a ride and perhaps threatened not to like her or talk to her if she didn't give in. Then she would be able to weigh the difficulty of dealing with her friends being angry at her against the difficulty of not being able to drive for several years.

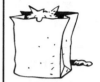

Consequences for breaking rules must be specific and concrete.

Summary

There are many ways to apply this *power struggle model* to different situations. It can be useful in dealing with children at home and at school. It can be applied to friends and co-workers because it is based on the fact that everyone controls only their own behavior. It helps us focus energy on things we can control and to treat

Properly using the power struggle model will make your life more safe and more sane no matter how other people are acting.

others with respect. It helps us to remember that a strong emotional response is a roadblock to getting what we need. This plan reminds us that we cannot make anyone do anything they don't want to do. They will either: do it when they are ready or do it when they feel the consequences outweigh the behavior. One of the most important parts of any plan like this is whether or not people have come to believe that *you will do what you say.* You must take steps to improve your credibility. The only way I know of doing this is to work a little at a time to only say things that you know you can and will do. After a while, you become believable and that in itself can make your life more safe, more sane and more comfortable, regardless of other people's behavior.

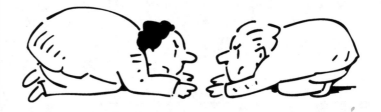

Practice Your Power Struggle Skills

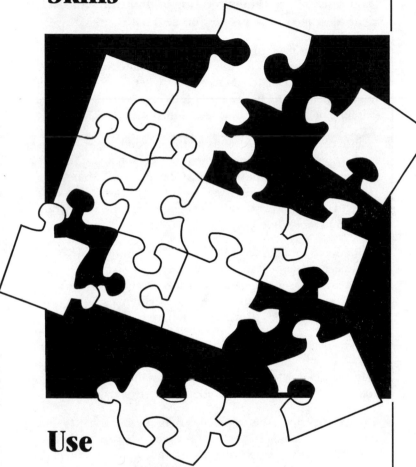

Use Yesterday's Power Struggle to Avoid One Today and Tomorrow

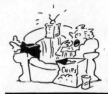

Use these charts to help visualize what needs to be done and help keep track of your progress.

Sending a Clear Message

Make a list of the things you can do that will help send a clear message to the people you deal with.

The following page provides a place to brainstorm or make a list of things that you think will communicate to the people in your life, how strongly you feel about what is acceptable and not acceptable. **The hardest part is to stop focusing on things you have no power over, including other people's behavior.**

Realize that the purpose of using things you have control over, is to send a clear message to the other person about just how strongly you feel about their behavior. This is not something you are trying to use to change the other person, but something that will make you feel as though you have done your job as a parent while keeping the situation safe and sane.

Write down things over which you have control, that you can use to get someone's attention when they don't do what you ask them to do. For your children, this can be anything as simple as permission to use a toy, or as complicated as losing a series of privileges that they then have to earn back.

With teenagers it may be more difficult to think of things you can do which will cause the person to stop and take notice of your message. The real focus for you should be how your actions reinforce your words about how strongly you feel.

The biggest trap in this situation is to try to find a way to change the teenager. Remember: teenagers are often masters of power struggles simply because they automatically focus on themselves and what they will do, right now, to get what they want.

With someone who is your equal or your partner, it may be even more difficult at first to think of things that will communicate how strongly you feel. Here, one of the biggest traps is to think of how to hurt or punish the other person. Instead, it might be useful to think about the positive aspects of your relationship with the other person. Then you can list the positive things you do in the relationship, which you will stop doing, if the other person refuses to do what you have asked them to do, or stop doing.

Think about what you can use to clearly communicate to others how strongly you feel.

Children

Privileges/Praise

_____

_____

_____

_____

Teenagers

Going out with friends/Use of the car/Spending money

_____

_____

_____

_____

_____

Adults

Affection/Housework/Laundry/Meals/Cooperation

_____

_____

_____

_____

_____

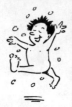

Describe how you can use the behaviors you listed in ways that fit the power struggle model.

On the following page, list how you can use the things **you have control over,** to make them fit the power struggle model's four rules. All four rules must be used at the same time for it to work.

Rule 1 - Describe how you can do the things listed.

Rule 2 - Describe anything you think might prevent you from following through on doing the things listed and ways you can remind yourself to follow through and do those things you say you will do.

Rule 3 - Describe the logic behind your decision to do these things to make sure that you are doing them without strong emotion.

Rule 4 - Describe how the things you have chosen to do will make your life better, safer, more sane, regardless of what other people choose to do.

If there are things you want to use in the power struggle facing you but they don't fit all four steps, how can you make changes in what you are doing or how you are doing it so that it follows all four steps.

Make a List, Follow These Simple Rules, Solve a Problem!

Use your own examples to personalize your list.

Rule 1 - Something you CAN do

_____
_____
_____
_____
_____

Rule 2 - Something you WILL do

_____
_____
_____
_____
_____

Rule 3 - Something you WILL DO WITHOUT strong emotion

_____
_____
_____
_____
_____

Rule 4 - You can't make others do anything they don't want to do. What can YOU do to make life better for YOU no matter what the other person does?

_____
_____
_____
_____
_____

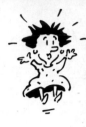

Practice your power struggle skills.

On the following page there is a chart to use to help you track your progress and skills at resolving power struggles.

In the first area, you should write something that helps you remember what the situation was that resulted in a power struggle.

In the next area, you should write what things you did to try to win, get out of, or resolve the power struggle.

In the area at the bottom, write down possible alternatives to use the next time a similar situation arises. The things you put in this area should follow all four rules of the power struggle model.

Use yesterday's power struggle to avoid one tomorrow!

The power struggle...

_____

_____

_____

_____

_____

_____

_____

What I did then...

_____

_____

_____

_____

_____

_____

_____

What I could have done...

_____

_____

_____

_____

_____

_____

_____

_____

Notes

50

ISBN 141203624-0